Keto Brea

Over 50 Easy Ketogenic Recipes To Start Your Day With A Big Smile

Kaylee LOPEZ

Table of Content

Coconut Cereal

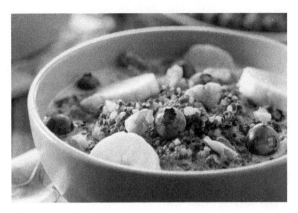

Servings: 16

Preparation time: 19 minutes Cooking time: 25

minutes

INGREDIENTS

- 1 tablespoon ground cinnamon 1 teaspoon ground nutmeg
- 1 tablespoon plus organic vanilla extract

  ½ teaspoon powdered stevia
- ½ cup water 1 pound unsweetened coconut flakes

DIRECTIONS

1. Preheat the oven to 300 degrees F. Line 3 cookie sheets with parchment paper.
2. In a large bowl, add all ingredients except coconut flakes and beat until well combined.
3. Transfer the coconut flakes in prepared cookie sheets evenly.

4. Bake for about 15 minutes.

5. Remove the cookie sheets from oven and stir the flakes.

6. Bake for 5-10 minutes more.

7. Remove from the oven and let it cool completely.

8. You can enjoy this cereal with any non-dairy milk and fruit's topping.

Meal Prep Tip: Transfer this cereal into an airtight container and preserve iin the refrigerator for 1-2 weeks.

NUTRITION: Net Carbs: 2.6g; Calories: 217; Total Fat: 19g; Sat. Fat: 16.6g; Protein: 2.4g; Carbs: 7.6g; Fiber: 5g; Sugar: 2.5g

Flax Seeds Bread

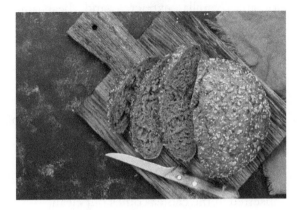

Servings: 12

Preparation time: 15 minutes Cooking

time: 28 minutes

INGREDIENTS

- 2 cups flax seeds meal 2 tablespoons Swerve

- 1 tablespoon organic baking powder ½ teaspoon salt

- 5 organic eggs, beaten 5 tablespoons butter, melted

- ½ cup water 1 teaspoon organic vanilla extract

DIRECTIONS

1. Preheat the oven to 350 degrees F. Line a 15x10-inch bread loaf pan with a lightly greased parchment paper.

2. In a large bowl, mix together the flax seeds meal, Swerve, baking powder and salt.

9

3. In another bowl, add the eggs, butter, water and organic vanilla extract and beat until well combined.

4. Add egg mixture into the bowl with flax seeds meal mixture and mix until well combined.

5. Transfer the bread mixture into prepared loaf pan evenly.

6. Bake for about 24-28 minutes or until a toothpick inserted in the center comes out clean.

7. Remove the bread pan from oven and keep onto a wire rack to cool for about 10 minutes.

8. Carefully invert the bread onto the wire rack to cool completely before serving.

9. With a sharp knife, cut the bread loaf in desired sized slices and serve.

10. Meal Prep Tip: In a reseal able plastic bag, place the bread slices and seal the bag after squeezing the excess air. Keep the bread away from direct sunlight and preserve in a cool and dryplace for about 1-2 days.

NUTRITION: Net Carbs: 2.8g; Calories: 196; Total Fat: 14.6g; Sat. Fat: 4.5g; Protein: 7.7g; Carbs: 9.1g; Fiber: 6.3g; Sugar: 0.2g

Blueberry Almond Plates

Servings: 4

Preparation time: 10 minutes Cooking time:

15 minutes

INGREDIENTS

- 1-½ cups almond flour
- ½ teaspoon baking powder
- 1-cup fresh blueberries
- 2 pastured eggs
- 2 tablespoon almond milk
- 2 tablespoons butter
- 2 tablespoons egg white
- ½ cup sliced almonds
- ¾ teaspoon cinnamon

DIRECTIONS

1. Melt butter over medium heat then let it cool.

2. Preheat an oven to 350°F (177°C and line a baking tray with parchment paper. Set aside.

3. Next, combine egg whites with sliced almond and cinnamon then stir well.

4. Place almond flour and baking powder in a mixing bowl then pour almond milk and melted butter over the dry mixture.

5. Add eggs to the mixture then mix until incorporated.

6. After that, stir fresh blueberries into the mixture then mix until just combined.

7. Divide the mixture into 4 balls then press until becoming approximately ½ inch thick circle.

8. Arrange on the prepared baking tray and top with the almond and cinnamon mixture.

9. Bake for approximately 15 minutes or lightly golden brown.

10. Once it is done, remove from the oven and let them cool.

11. Serve and enjoy.

NUTRITION: Net Carbs: 6.7g; Calories: 253; Total Fat: 21.1g; Sat. Fat: 6.8g; Protein: 9.1g; Carbs: 10.4g; Fiber: 3.7g; Sugar: 3.9g

Zucchini Pancakes

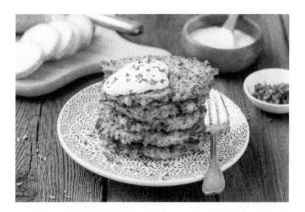

Servings: 6

Preparation time: 15 minutes Cooking

time: 36 minutes

INGREDIENTS

- 2 medium zucchinis, grated and squeezed 2 organic eggs
- 1 ounce almond meal Salt and ground black pepper, as required
- 2 tablespoons coconut oil

DIRECTIONS

- In a bowl, add all the ingredients except the coconut oil and mix well.
- Set aside for about 4-5 minutes.
- In a large skillet, melt coconut oil over medium heat.

- Add the desired amount of the zucchini mixture and cook for about 2-3 minutes per side.

- Repeat with the remaining mixture.

- Serve warm.

Meal Prep Tip: Store these cooled pancakes into an airtight container by placing a piece of wax paper between each pancake. Refrigerate up to 4 days. Reheat in the microwave for about 1½-2 minutes.

NUTRITION: Net Carbs: 2.2g; Calories: 144; Total Fat: 11.5g; Sat. Fat: 6.9g; Protein: 8.2g; Carbs: 3.5g; Fiber: 1.3g; Sugar: 1.4g

Keto Brunch Spread

Preparation Time: 10minutes

Cooking Time: 20 Minutes Serving: 4

INGREDIENTS

- 4 large eggs
- 24 asparagus spears
- 12 slices of pastured, sugar-free bacon

DIRECTIONS

1. Pre-warmness your range to 400F

2. At that point, two with the aid of, wrap them with one reduce of bacon. Hold your lances immovably and close to one another with one hand as you wind the reduce of bacon beginning from the base, to the highest factor of the lance.

3. A spot in the range set the clock for 20mins.

4. In this time, bring a little pot of water to a fast bubble. Tenderly vicinity 4 big eggs inside the effervescent water, set any other clock for 6mins.

5. At the factor when the 6mins are up, make use of an opened spoon or tongs to unexpectedly move your eggs to the ice shower, let them take a seat for 2mins before stripping the finishes off.

6. Delicately ruin the highest factor of the egg on a hard surface and strip away the shell to discover the tip of the egg.

7. At the point whilst the asparagus is ready, serve on a plate or cutting board. In the occasion that you do not have an egg holder use coffee cups to maintain your eggs up.

8. Dunk your asparagus lances into your eggs. Gala, recognize it!

NUTRITION: Calories: 426, Fat 38g, Carbs 3g, Sugar 3g, Protein 17g

Meat-Lover Pizza Cups

Preparation Time: 15minutes Cooking Time: 11

Minutes Serving: 12

INGREDIENTS

- 12 deli ham slices
- 1 lb. bulk Italian sausage
- 12 Tbsp sugar-free pizza sauce
- 3 cups grated mozzarella cheese
- 24 pepperoni slices
- 1 cup cooked and crumbled bacon

DIRECTIONS

- Preheat broiler to 375 F. Dark-colored Italian frankfurters in a skillet, depleting abundance oil.
- Line 12-cup biscuit tin with ham cuts. Partition wiener, pizza sauce, mozzarella cheddar, pepperoni cuts, and bacon disintegrate between each cup, in a specific order.
- Heat at 375 for 10 minutes, cook for 1 moment until cheddar air pockets and tans and the edges of the meat ingredients look firm.
-
- Remove pizza cups from biscuit tin and set on a paper towels

to keep the bottoms from getting wet. Appreciate promptly or refrigerate and warm in toaster stove or microwave.

NUTRITION: Calories 165, Fat 14g, Carbs 11g, Sugar 2g, Protein 2g

White Lasagna Stuffed Peppers

Preparation Time: 5minutes

Cooking Time: 1hr Serving: 4

INGREDIENTS

- 2 large sweet peppers
- 1 tsp garlic salt
- 12 oz ground turkey
- 3/4 cup ricotta cheese
- 1 cup mozzarella

DIRECTIONS

1. Preheat stove to 40
2. Put the split peppers in a heating dish. Sprinkle with 1/4 tsp garlic salt. Gap the ground turkey between the peppers and press into the bottoms. Sprinkle with another 1/4 tsp garlic salt. Prepare for 30 minutes.
3. Partition the ricotta cheddar between the peppers. Sprinkle with the staying 1/2 tsp garlic salt. Sprinkle the mozzarella on top. Put the cherry tomatoes in the middle of the peppers, if utilizing.

4. Prepare for an extra 30 minutes until the peppers are mollified, the meat is cooked, and the cheddar is

brilliant.

NUTRITION: Calories 281, Fat 14g, Carbs 7g, Sugars 1g, Protein 32g

Easy Taco Casserole Recipe

Preparation Time: 5minutes Cooking Time: 40 Minutes Serving: 6

INGREDIENTS

- 2 lb ground turkey or beef
- 2 tbsp taco seasoning
- 1 cup of salsa
- 16 oz cottage cheese
- 8 oz shredded cheddar cheese

DIRECTIONS

1. Preheat range to four hundred.
2. Blend the ground meat and taco flavoring in a massive goulash dish. Heat for 20mins
3. In the interim, combine the curds, salsa, and 1 cup of the cheddar. Put in a safe spot.
4. Remove the meal dish from the broiler and cautiously channel the cooking fluid from the meat.
5. Separate the beef into little portions. A potato masher works first-rate for this. Spread the curds and salsa mixture over the beef.
6. Return the meal to the broiler and heat for a further 15-20 minutes till the meat is cooked all collectively and the cheddar

is warm and bubbly.

NUTRITION: Calories 367, Fat 18g, Carbs 6g, Sugars 4g, Protein 45g

Cold Brew Protein Shake Smoothie

Preparation Time: 10 Minutes Serving: 1

INGREDIENTS

- 8 oz cold brew coffee
- 1/3 cup almond milk
- 1 scoop Rootz Paleo Chocolate Banana
- A handful of ice cubes

DIRECTIONS

1. Join all Ingredients in milk frothier or a shaker bottle. Blend until very much consolidated.

NUTRITION: Calories 188; Fat 5g, Carbs 10g, Sugar 6g, Protein 24g

Ricotta Pancakes

Servings: 4

Preparation time: 15 minutes

Cooking time: 21 minutes

INGREDIENTS

- 4 organic eggs ½ cup ricotta cheese
- ¼ cup vanilla whey protein powder ½ teaspoon organic baking powder
- Pinch of salt ½ teaspoon liquid stevia
- 2 tablespoons butter

DIRECTIONS

1. In a blender, add all the Ingredients and pulse until well combined.
2. In a skillet, melt the butter over medium heat.
3. Add the desired amount of the mixture and spread it evenly.
4. Cook for about 2-3 minutes or until golden brown.
5. Flip and cook for about 1-2 minutes or until golden brown.
6. Repeat with the remaining mixture.
7. Serve warm.

Meal Prep Tip: Store these cooled pancakes in an airtight container by placing a piece of wax paper between each pancake. Refrigerate up to 4 days. Reheat in the microwave for about 1½-2 minutes.

NUTRITION: Net Carbs: 1.6; Calories: 124; Total Fat: 8.7g; Sat. Fat: 4.5g; Protein: 4.4g; Carbs: 1.6g; Fiber: 0g; Sugar: 0.5g

Cream Cheese Pancakes

Servings: 3

Preparation time: 15 minutes

Cooking time: 6 minutes

INGREDIENTS

- 2 large organic eggs 2 ounces cream cheese, softened
- 1/3 teaspoon organic baking powder 1/3 teaspoon ground cinnamon
- ½ teaspoon organic vanilla extract 2-3 drops liquid stevia

DIRECTIONS

1. In a blender, add all the Nutritional Info per Serving: and pulse until smooth.
2. Set aside for about 2-3 minutes.
3. Heat a greased nonstick skillet over medium heat.
4. Add ¼ of the mixture and with a spoon, spread it.
5. Cook for 2 minutes or until golden brown.
6. Flip and cook for about 1 minute.
7. Repeat with the remaining mixture.
8. Serve warm.

Meal Prep Tip: Store these cooled pancakes in an airtight container by placing a piece of wax paper between each pancake. Refrigerate up to 4 days. Reheat in the microwave for about 1½-2 minutes.

NUTRITION: Net Carbs: 1.1g; Calories: 117; Total Fat: 9.9g; Sat. Fat: 5.2g; Protein: 5.6g; Carbs: 1.3g; Fiber: 0.2g; Sugar: 0.4g

Tomato Beef Bagels

Servings: 4

Preparation time: 5 minutes Cooking
time: 35 minutes

INGREDIENTS

- 1 lb. ground beef
  - ¾ cup diced onion
  - 1-tablespoon butter
  - 2 pastured eggs
  - ½ cup tomato puree
  - 1 ½ teaspoon paprika
  - ½ teaspoon salt
  - ¾ teaspoon pepper

DIRECTIONS

1. Preheat an oven to 400°F (204°C and line a baking tray with parchment paper. Set aside.

2. Next, preheat a saucepan over medium heat and place butter in it.

3. Once the butter is melted, stir in diced onion and sauté until wilted and aromatic. Remove from heat and let it cool.

4. When the sautéed onion is cool, add ground beef together with eggs and tomato puree then season with paprika, salt, and pepper. Mix until combined.

5. Shape the beef mixture into 8 medium bagel forms then arrange on the prepared baking tray.

6. Bake the beef bagels for approximately 35 minutes or until the beef bagels are completely cooked.

7. Once it is done, remove the cooked beef bagels from the oven and let it warm.

8. Place 4 bagels on a serving dish then put sliced tomatoes, onion, lettuce, cheese, or any kinds of burger filling, as you desired.

9. Top with the remaining beef bagels then serve immediately. Enjoy!

NUTRITION: Net Carbs: 4.3g; Calories: 415; Total Fat: 33.3g; Sat. Fat: 13.6g; Protein: 21.9g; Carbs: 5.7g; Fiber: 1.4g; Sugar: 2.5g

-

Bacon Omelet

Servings: 2

Preparation time: 15 minutes

Cooking time: 15 minutes

INGREDIENTS

- 4 large organic eggs 1 tablespoon fresh chives, minced
- Salt and ground black pepper, as required 4 bacon slices
- 1 tablespoon unsalted butter 2 ounces Cheddar cheese, shredded

DIRECTIONS

1. In a bowl, add the eggs, chives, salt and black pepper and beat until well combined.
2. Heat a non-stick frying pan over medium- high heat and cook the bacon slices for about 8-10 minutes.
3. Place the bacon onto a paper towel-lined plate to drain. Then chop the bacon slices.
4. With paper towels, wipe out the frying pan.
5. In the same frying pan, melt the butter over medium-low heat and cook the egg mixture for about 2 minutes.

6. Carefully, flip the omelet and top with chopped bacon.

7. Cook for 1-2 minutes or until desired doneness of eggs.

8. Remove from heat and immediately, place the cheese in the center of omelet.

9. Fold the edges of omelet over cheese and cut into 2 portions.

10. Serve immediately.

NUTRITION: Net Carbs: 2g; Calories: 633; Total Fat: 49.3g; Sat. Fat: 20.7g; Protein: 41.2 g; Carbs: 2g; Fiber: 0g; Sugar: 1g

Poppy Seeds Muffins

Servings: 12

Preparation time: 15 minutes

Cooking time: 20 minutes

INGREDIENTS

- ¾ cup blanched almond flour ¼ cup golden flax meal
- 1/3 cup Erythritol 2 tablespoons poppy seeds
- 1 teaspoon organic baking powder 3 large organic eggs
- ¼ cup heavy cream ¼ cup salted butter, melted
- 3 tablespoons fresh lemon juice 1 teaspoon organic vanilla extract
- 8-10 drops liquid stevia 2 teaspoons fresh lemon zest, grated finely

DIRECTIONS

1. Preheat the oven to 350 degrees F. Line 12 cups of a muffin tin with paper liners.
2. In a large bowl, add the flour, flax meal, poppy seeds, Erythritol and baking powder and mix well.
3. In another bowl, add the eggs, heavy cream and butter and beat until well combined.
4. Add the egg mixture into the flour mixture and mix until well combined and smooth.
5. Add the lemon juice, organic vanilla extract and liquid stevia

and mix until well combined.

6. Gently, fold in lemon zest.

7. Transfer the mixture into prepared muffin cups evenly.

8. Bake for about 18-20 minutes or until a toothpick inserted in the center comes out clean.

9. Remove the muffin tin from oven and place onto a wire rack to cool for about 10 minutes.

10. Carefully invert the muffins onto a wire rack to cool completely before serving.

Meal Prep Tip: Carefully invert the muffins onto a wire rack to cool completely. Line 1-2 airtight containers with paper towels. Arrange muffins over paper towel in a single layer. Cover muffins with another paper towel. Refrigerate for about

2-4 days. Reheat in the microwave on High for about 2 minutes before serving.

NUTRITION: Net Carbs: 1.6g; Calories: 124; Total Fat: 10.9g; Sat. Fat: 3.8g; Protein: 4g; Carbs: 3.2g; Fiber: 1.6g; Sugar: 0.4g

Vanilla Cream Pancakes

Servings: 4

Preparation time: 15 minutes

Cooking time: 20 minutes

INGREDIENTS

- ½ cup almond flour, sifted ¼ teaspoon organic baking powder
- 2ouncesheavy whipping cream 2large organic eggs, separated
- 2teaspoons granulated Erythritol Pinch of salt
- 2teaspoonsunsalted butter

DIRECTIONS

1. In a bowl, add the flour and baking powder and mix well.
2. In another bowl, add the whipping cream, egg yolks, Erythritol and salt and beat until smooth.
3. Add the flour mixture and mix until well combined.
4. In a clean glass bowl, add the egg whites with an electric mixer, beat until soft peaks form.
5. Add the whipped egg whites into the bowl of nuts mixture and gently, stir to combine.
6. In a large non-stick frying pan, melt ½ teaspoon of

butter over medium heat.

7. Add ¼ of the mixture and with a spoon, spread it.

8. Cook for 3 minutes or until golden brown.

9. Flip and cook for about 2 minutes or until golden brown.

10. Repeat with the remaining mixture.

11. Serve warm.

NUTRITION: Net Carbs: 2.2g; Calories: 182; Total Fat: 16.6g; Sat. Fat: 15.8g; Protein: 6.5g; Carbs: 3.7g; Fiber: 1.5g; Sugar: 0.7g

Spicy Green Omelets

Servings: 4

Preparation time: 5 minutes

Cooking time: 15 minutes

INGREDIENTS

- 8 pastured eggs
- ½ cup diced green bell peppers
- ¼ cup cooked green peas
- ¼ cup chopped onion
- 2 tablespoons chopped leek
- 1 teaspoon sliced shallots
- 1 teaspoon chopped green chili
- ¼ cup diced cheddar cheese
- ¼ cup coconut milk
- 2 tablespoons extra virgin olive oil

DIRECTIONS

9. Crack the eggs and place in a bowl. Stir until beaten.
10. Add chopped green bell pepper, cooked green peas, chopped onion, chopped leek, sliced shallots, green chili, and cheddar cheese to the bowl.
11. Pour coconut milk over the eggs then mix until combined.

Set aside.

12. Preheat a saucepan over medium heat then pour extra virgin olive oil into the saucepan.

13. Once it is hot, pour the egg mixture over the saucepan and spread evenly.

14. Cook the omelet for approximately 3-5 minutes or until the eggs are firm.

15. Remove the omelet from the saucepan and transfer to a serving dish.

16. Serve and enjoy.

NUTRITION: Net Carbs: 5.1g: Calories: 284; Total Fat: 22.4g; Sat. Fat: 8.9g; Protein: 15.2g; Carbs: 6.4g; Fiber: 1.3g; Sugar: 1.9g

-

Chicken Frittata

Servings: 4

Preparation time: 15 minutes

Cooking time: 12 minutes

INGREDIENTS

- ½ cup grass-fed cooked chicken, chopped 1/3 cup Parmesan cheese, grated
- 6 organic eggs, beaten lightly
- Salt and ground black pepper, as required 1 teaspoon butter
- ½ cup boiled asparagus, chopped 1 tablespoon fresh parsley, chopped

DIRECTIONS

- Preheat the broiler of oven.
- In a bowl, add the cheese, eggs, salt and black pepper and beat until well combined.
- In a large ovenproof skillet, melt the butter over medium-high heat and cook the chicken and asparagus for about 2-3 minutes.
- Add the egg mixture and stir to combine,
- Cook for about 4-5 minutes.

- Remove from the heat and sprinkle with parsley.

- Now, transfer the skillet under broiler and broil for about 3-4 minutes or until slightly puffed.

- Cut into desired sized wedges and serve immediately.

Meal Prep Tip: In a resealable plastic bag, place the cooled frittata slices and seal the bag. Refrigerate for about 2-4 days. Reheat in the microwave on High for about 1 minute before serving.

NUTRITION: Net Carbs: 2.2g; Calories: 213; Total Fat: 13.4g; Sat. Fat: 6.2g; Protein: 21.8g; Carbs: 2.6g; Fiber: 0.4g; Sugar: 21.8g

Sunny Side Up in Bell Pepper Bowls

Servings: 4

Preparation time: 5 minutes

Cooking time: 15 minutes

INGREDIENTS

- 2 bell peppers
- 8 pastured eggs
- ¼ teaspoon salt
- ¼ teaspoon peppers
- 3 tablespoons chopped parsley
- ¼ cup butter
- Place 2 tablespoons of butter in a saucepan over medium heat then wait until melted.

DIRECTIONS

1. Once the butter is melted, cut a bell pepper into 4 rings then place in the saucepan.
2. Drop an egg in each bell pepper ring then sprinkle salt, pepper, and chopped parsley on top. Cook for approximately 4 minutes or until the egg is set.
3. Once it is done, remove the bell peppers with sunny side up from the saucepan and arrange on a serving dish.
4. Repeat with the remaining bell peppers, eggs, and seasoning then arrange them all on a serving dish.

5. Serve and enjoy warm.

6. If you like, you can also sprinkle paprika over the eggs.

NUTRITION: Net Carbs: 6.1g; Calories: 319; Total Fat: 25.3g; Sat. Fat: 13.2g; Protein: 16.4g; Carbs: 7g; Fiber: 0.9g; Sugar: 3.1g

Cheddar Waffles

Servings: 8

Preparation time: 15 minutes

Cooking time: 48 minutes

INGREDIENTS

- 1 cup golden flax seeds meal 1 cup almond flour

- ¼ cup unflavored whey protein powder 2 teaspoons organic baking powder

- Salt and ground black pepper, as required 1½ cups cheddar cheese, shredded

- ¾ cup unsweetened almond milk ¼ cup unsalted butter, melted

- 4 large organic eggs, beaten

DIRECTIONS

1. Preheat the waffle iron and then grease it.

2. In a large bowl, add flax seeds meal, flour, protein powder and baking powder and mix well.

3. Stir in the cheddar cheese.

4. In another bowl, add remaining ingredients and beat until well combined.

5. Add the egg mixture into the bowl of flax seeds meal mixture and mix until well combined.

6. Place the desired amount of the mixture into preheated waffle iron.

7. Cook for about 4-6 minutes or until golden brown.

8. Repeat with the remaining mixture.

9. Serve warm.

NUTRITION: Net Carbs: 4.1g; Calories: 365; Total Fat: 28.6g; Sat. Fat: 10.1g; Protein: 19.1g; Carbs: 10.4g; Fiber: 6.3g; Sugar: 0.8g

Cauliflower Almond Fritters with Lemon Creamy Sauce

Servings: 4

Preparation time: 10 minutes

Cooking time: 15 minutes

INGREDIENTS

- 2 cups cauliflower florets
- ¼ cup diced onion
- 2 pastured eggs
- ½ cup almond flour
- ½ teaspoon turmeric
- ½ teaspoon salt
- ¼ teaspoon pepper
- ½ teaspoon garlic powder
- 2 tablespoons butter
- Coconut oil, to fry
- 3 egg yolks
- 2 tablespoons lemon juice
- ¼ teaspoon paprika

DIRECTIONS

1. Place the cauliflower florets in a pot then pour water to cover. Bring to boil.

2. Once it is boiled, reduce the heat and cook the cauliflower florets for about 5 minutes.

3. Remove the pot from heat and strain the cauliflower.

4. Transfer the cooked cauliflower to a food processor and pulse until becoming rice form.

5. Place the cauliflower rice in a bowl then add diced onion, eggs and almond flour.

6. Season the cauliflower mixture with turmeric, salt, pepper, and garlic powder then mix well.

7. Shape the cauliflower mixture into 4 medium fritters then set aside.

8. Melt butter in a saucepan over medium heat then place the cauliflower fritters in the saucepan.

9. Cook the cauliflower florets for approximately 3 minutes each side or until both sides of the cauliflower fritters are lightly golden brown.

10. In the meantime, pour hot water into a blender and let it sit for 10 minutes.

11. Next, preheat the coconut oil to approximately 95°F (35°C then set aside.

12. After 10 minutes, discard the water from the blender and place egg yolks and lemon juice into the hot blender.

13. Pour hot coconut oil over the egg yolks then season with paprika. Blend the sauce mixture on low until incorporated.

14. Arrange the cauliflower fritters on a serving dish then drizzle the sauce on top.

15. Serve and enjoy.

NUTRITION: Net Carbs: 3.8g: Calories: 284; Total Fat: 26.9g; Sat. Fat: 17.6g; Protein: 7.1g; Carbs: 5.8g; Fiber: 2g; Sugar: 2g -

Chocolate Pancakes

Preparation time: 15 minutes

Cooking time: 16 minutes

INGREDIENTS

- 4tablespoonscoconut   flour
  2teaspoonsorganic baking powder
- 2 teaspoons xylitol Pinch of salt
- 4 ounces cream cheese, softened 3 organic eggs
- 1 tablespoon organic vanilla extract ¼ cup 70% dark chocolate chips
- 2-3 tablespoons unsweetened almond milk

DIRECTIONS

1. In a blender, add all the ingredients except the almond milk and pulse until creamy and smooth.
2. Set aside for about 5 minutes.
3. Again, pulse for about 10 seconds.
4. Now, add almond milk and pulse until well combined.
5. Heat a lightly greased nonstick skillet over medium heat.
6. Add 1/3 cup of mixture and cook for about 2 minutes or until golden brown.
7. Flip and cook for about 1-2 minutes.
8. Repeat with the remaining mixture.

9. Serve warm.

NUTRITION: Net Carbs: 6g; Calories: 291; Total Fat: 22g; Sat. Fat: 12.8g; Protein: 9.3g; Carbs: 11.1g; Fiber: 5.1g; Sugar: 0.7g

Veggie Quiche

Servings: 4

Preparation time: 15 minutes

Cooking time: 20 minutes

INGREDIENTS

- 6 organic eggs ½ cup unsweetened almond milk
- Salt and ground black pepper, as required 1 cup fresh baby spinach, chopped
- 1 cup fresh baby kale, chopped ½ cup bell pepper, seeded and chopped
- 1 scallion, chopped ¼ cup fresh cilantro, chopped
- 1 tablespoon fresh chives, minced 3 tablespoons mozzarella cheese, grated

DIRECTIONS

1. Preheat the oven to 400 degrees F (200 C. Lightly grease a pie dish.
2. In a large bowl, add the eggs, almond milk, salt and black pepper and beat until well combined.
3. Set aside.
4. In another bowl, add the vegetables and herbs and mix well.
5. In the bottom of prepared pie dish, place the veggie mixture evenly and top with the egg mixture.
6. Bake for about 20 minutes or until a wooden skewer inserted in the center comes out clean.

7. Remove from the oven and immediately sprinkle with the Parmesan cheese.

8. Set aside for about 5 minutes before serving.

9. Cut into desired sized wedges and serve warm.

NUTRITION: Net Carbs: 4.1g; Calories: 176; Total Fat: 10.9g; Sat. Fat: 4.3g; Protein: 15.4g; Carbs: 5g; Fiber: 0.9g; Sugar: 1.4g

Chocolate Muffins

Servings: 12

Preparation time: 15 minutes

Cooking time: 20 minutes

INGREDIENTS

- 1 cup almond flour ½ cup Erythritol
- ½ cup cacao powder 1½ teaspoons organic baking powder
- ¼ teaspoon salt 2/3 cup heavy cream
- 3 ounces unsalted butter, melted 3 organic eggs
- 1 teaspoon organic vanilla extract ½ cup 70% dark chocolate chips

DIRECTIONS

1. Preheat the oven to 350 degrees F. Line 12 cups of a muffin tin with paper liners.
2. In a large bowl, add the flour, Erythritol, cacao powder, baking powder and salt and mix well.
3. In another bowl, add the heavy cream, butter, eggs and vanilla extract and beat until well combined.
4. Place the egg mixture into the bowl of flour mixture and mix until just blended.
5. Gently, fold in the chocolate chips.
6. Place the mixture into each prepared muffin cup evenly.

7. Bake for about 20 minutes or until a toothpick inserted in the center comes out clean.

8. Remove the muffin tin from oven and place onto a wire rack to cool for about 10 minutes.

9. Carefully invert the muffins onto a wire rack to cool completely before serving.

Meal Prep Tip: Carefully invert the muffins onto a wire rack to cool completely. Line 1-2 airtight containers with paper towels. Arrange muffins over paper towel in a single layer. Cover muffins with another paper towel. Refrigerate for about 2-3 days. Reheat in the microwave on High for about 2 minutes before serving.

NUTRITION: Net Carbs: 4g; Calories: 176; Total Fat: 16g; Sat. Fat: 7.1g; Protein: 4.6g; Carbs: 6g; Fiber: 2g; Sugar: 4.1g

1. Coconut Nutty Granola Bars with Cranberries

Servings: 4

Preparation time: 5 minutes

Cooking time: 20 minutes

INGREDIENTS

- ½ cup coconut flakes
- ¼ cup sliced roasted almonds
- 2 tablespoons chopped roasted pecans
- ¼ cup chopped roasted cashews
- ¼ cup sunflower seeds
- ½ cup chopped dried cranberries
- ¼ teaspoon salt
- ½ cup almond butter
- 2 teaspoons olive oil

DIRECTIONS

1. Place almond butter in a microwave-safe bowl then microwave until melted. Let it cool.
2. Preheat an oven to 300°F (149°C and line a small square baking pan with parchment paper. Set aside.
3. Place coconut flakes, roasted almonds, roasted pecans,

roasted cashews, salt, and sunflower seeds in a food processor then process until becoming crumbles. Transfer to a mixing bowl.

4. Pour melted butter and olive oil over the crumbles then mix until combined.

5. Transfer the mixture to the prepared baking pan then press evenly.

6. Bake the granola for approximately 20 minutes or until the top of the granola is lightly golden brown.

7. Once it is done, remove the granola from the oven and let it cool for a few minutes.

8. Using a very sharp knife cut the granola into bars and arrange on a serving dish.

9. Serve and enjoy!

NUTRITION: Net Carbs: 5.5g: Calories: 276; Total Fat: 25.7g; Sat. Fat: 5.4g; Protein: 5.3g; Carbs: 9.7g; Fiber: 4.2g; Sugar: 2.5g

2. Turkey Hash

Servings: 5

Preparation time: 15 minutes

Cooking time: 20 minutes

INGREDIENTS

- 3 cups cauliflower florets 2 tablespoons unsalted butter

- 1 small yellow onion, chopped 1 teaspoon dried thyme, crushed

- Salt and ground black pepper, as required 1 pound cooked turkey meat, chopped

- ¼ cup heavy cream

DIRECTIONS

1. In a pan of salted boiling water, add the cauliflower and cook for about 4 minutes.

2. Drain the cauliflower well and rinse under cold running water.

3. Then chop the cauliflower and set aside.

4. In a large skillet, melt the butter over medium heat and sauté onion for about 4-5 minutes.

5. Add thyme, salt and black pepper and sauté for about 1 minute.

6. Stir in cauliflower and cook for about 2 minutes.

7. Stir in turkey and cook for about 5-6 minutes.

8. Stir in the cream and cook for about 2 minutes more.

9. Serve warm.

Meal Prep Tip: Transfer the cooled scramble into airtight container and refrigerate for up to 3 days. Reheat in microwave before serving.

NUTRITION: Net Carbs: 2.9g; Calories: 237; Total Fat: 11.5g; Sat. Fat: 5.8g; Protein: 28.1g; Carbs: 4.8g; Fiber: 1.9g; Sugar: 2g

Choco Coconut Waffles

Preparation Time: 5 minutes Cooking Time: 3 minutes Servings: 1

INGREDIENTS

- 1 egg, lightly beaten
- 1 tsp coconut oil
- 2 tbsp water
- 1 tsp baking powder, gluten-free
- 1 tsp coconut flour
- 1 scoop chocolate protein powder
- 1/2 tsp vanilla

DIRECTIONS

1. Preheat the waffle iron.
2. Add all ingredients into the mixing bowl and whisk until well combined.
3. Spray waffle iron with cooking spray.
4. Pour batter onto hot iron and cook waffle until crisp.
5. Serve and enjoy.

NUTRITION: Calories 178 Fat 9.9 g Carbohydrates 6.6 g Sugar 1.6 g Protein 15.9 g

Cholesterol 184 mg

Egg Avocado Casserole

Preparation Time: 10 minutes Cooking Time: 4 hours

Servings: 8

INGREDIENTS

- 8 eggs, lightly beaten
- 1/2 cup unsweetened coconut milk
- 1 cup cheddar cheese, shredded
- 1 avocado, chopped
- Pepper
- Salt

DIRECTIONS

1. Spray slow cooker from inside with cooking spray.
2. Add all ingredients into the mixing bowl and whisk until well combined. Pour into the slow cooker.
3. Cover and cook on low for 4 hours.
4. Serve and enjoy.

NUTRITION: Calories 206 Fat 17.5 g Carbohydrates 3.5 g Sugar 1 g Protein 9.9 g

Cholesterol 179 mg

Spinach and Cheese Egg Muffins

Servings: 4

Preparation time: 5 minutes Cooking time: 15 minutes **INGREDIENTS**

- 8 pastured eggs
- 2 tablespoons butter
- 2 tablespoons chopped onion
- 1-cup chopped spinach
- ¼ teaspoon salt
- ½ teaspoon pepper
- 1-¼ cups grated Mozzarella cheese
- ½ cup grated cheddar cheese

DIRECTIONS

1. Preheat an oven to 400°F (204°C and prepare 8 medium muffin cups. Coat with cooking spray.

2. Next, preheat a skillet over medium heat and place butter in it. Wait until the butter is melted.

3. Stir in chopped onion then sauté until aromatic and lightly golden brown.

4. After that, add chopped spinach to the skillet and cook until the spinach is wilted but still green. Remove from heat and let it cool.

5. Divide the sautéed spinach and onion into the prepared

muffin cups then set aside.

6. Crack the eggs and place in a bowl.

7. Next, season the eggs with salt, pepper, and Mozzarella cheese. Stir until incorporated.

8. Pour the egg mixture over the spinach in the aluminum muffin cups then sprinkle grated cheddar cheese on top.

9. Bake the egg muffins for approximately 15-20 minutes or until the egg is firm.

10. Once the egg muffins are done, remove from the oven and let them rest for a few minutes.

11. Take the muffins out of the cups and arrange on a serving dish.

12. Serve and enjoy.

NUTRITION: Net Carbs: 3g: Calories: 385; Total Fat: 30.4g; Sat. Fat: 16.4g; Protein: 24.3g; Carbs: 3.7g; Fiber: 0.7g; Sugar: 0.4g -

Protein Smoothie

Servings: 2

Preparation time: 15 minutes

INGREDIENTS

- 1½ scoops unsweetened vanilla whey protein powder
- 4 tablespoons almond butter 3 tablespoons golden flax meal
- 15 drops liquid stevia 1/8 teaspoon organic vanilla extract
- 1¾ cups unsweetened nut milk

DIRECTIONS

1. In a blender, place all the ingredients and pulse until smooth.
2. Place the smoothie into glasses and serve immediately

Meal Prep Tip: In 2 mason jars, divide the smoothie. Seal the jars and freeze for 1-2 days. Before serving, thaw the smoothie. Just before serving, in each jar, add a splash of almond milk and stir well.

NUTRITION: Net Carbs: 2.2g; Calories: 364; Total Fat: 25.7g;

Sat. Fat: 1.9g; Protein: 26.5g; Carbs: 12g; Fiber: 7.3g; Sugar: 2.4g

Nuts Granola

Servings: 12

Preparation time: 15 minutes

Cooking time: 18 minutes

INGREDIENTS

- 1½ cups almonds 1½ cups hazelnuts
- ¼ cup cacao powder 1 cup flax seeds meal
- Pinch of sea salt ¼ cup hazelnut oil
- ¼ cup almond butter, melted 2 ounces 70% dark chocolate, chopped
- 1/3 cup Erythritol 20 drops stevia extract

DIRECTIONS

1. Preheat the oven to 300 degrees F. Line a large baking sheet with parchment paper.
2. In a food processor, add almonds and hazelnuts and pulse until a coarse crumb forms.
3. In a large bowl. place the nuts mixture.
4. Add the cacao powder, flax seeds meal and salt and mix well.
5. In a pan, add hazelnut oil, butter and chocolate over low heat and cook for about 2-3 minutes or until smooth, stirring continuously.

6. Stir in swerve and immediately, remove from heat.

7. Add butter mixture over nut mixture and toss to coat well.

8. Transfer the mixture onto prepared baking sheet evenly.

9. Bake for about 15 minutes, stirring after every 5 minutes.

10. Turn off the oven but keep the baking sheet in oven for about 20 minutes, stirring occasionally.

11. Remove from the oven and let it cool completely.

Meal Prep Tip: Transfer granola in an airtight container and store in a cool, dry place for up to 2 weeks.

NUTRITION: Net Carbs: 4.6g; Calories: 255; Total Fat: 21.2g; Sat. Fat: 2.2g; Protein: 7.9g; Carbs: 10.8g; Fiber: 6.2g; Sugar: 2.2g

Cheese Crepes

Servings: 5

Preparation time: 15 minutes Cooking time: 20 minutes **INGREDIENTS**

- 6 ounces cream cheese, softened 1/3cupParmesan cheese, grated
- 6 large organic eggs 1teaspoon Erythritol
- 1½ tablespoon coconut flour 1/8 teaspoon xanthan gum
- 2 tablespoons butter

DIRECTIONS

1. In a blender, add the cream cheese, Parmesan cheese, eggs and Erythritol and pulse on low speed until well combined.
2. While the motor is running, place the coconut flour and xanthan gum and pulse until a thick mixture is formed.
3. Now, pulse on medium speed for a few seconds.
4. Transfer the mixture into a bowl and set aside for about 5 minutes.
5. In a nonstick pan, melt the butter over medium-low heat.
6. Add ¼ cup of the mixture and tilt the pan to spread into

a thin layer.

7. Cook for about 1½ minutes or until the edges become brown.

8. Flip the crepe and cook for about 15-20 seconds more.

9. Repeat with the remaining mixture.

Meal Prep Tip: Keep the crepes aside to cool completely before storing. With a plastic wrap, cover the crepes and refrigerate up to 2 days. Reheat each crepe in the microwave for about 30 seconds.

NUTRITION: Net Carbs: 2.2g; Calories: 283; Total Fat: 24.3g; Sat. Fat: 13.5g; Protein: 12.9g; Carbs: 3.8g; Fiber: 1.6g; Sugar: 0.8g

Cauliflower Waffles

Servings: 4

Preparation time: 15 minutes

Cooking time: 23 minutes

INGREDIENTS

- 1½ cups cauliflower, grated   ½ cup cheddar cheese
- ½ cup mozzarella cheese ¼ cup Parmesan cheese
- 3 large organic eggs 3 tablespoons fresh chives, chopped
  - ¼ teaspoon red pepper flakes, crushed Salt and ground black pepper, as required

DIRECTIONS

1. In a food processor, add all the ingredients and pulse until well combined.
2. Preheat the waffle iron and then grease it.
3. Place desired amount of the mixture into preheated waffle iron and cook for about 7-10 minutes or until desired doneness.
4. Repeat with the remaining mixture.
5. Serve warm.

Meal Prep Tip: Store these waffles in an airtight container by placing a piece of wax paper between each waffle. Refrigerate up to 2-3 days. Reheat in the microwave for about 1-2 minutes.

NUTRITION: Net Carbs: 2.2g; Calories: 154; Total Fat: 10.5g; Sat. Fat: 5.4g; Protein: 12g; Carbs: 3.3g; Fiber: 1.1g; Sugar: 1.5g

Chicken Quiche

Servings: 8

Preparation time: 15 minutes Cooking time:

45 minutes

INGREDIENTS

- 2 cups grass-fed cooked chicken, chopped 1 teaspoon butter
- ½ cup yellow onion, sliced 2 garlic cloves, minced
- 3 cups small broccoli florets 2 large organic eggs
- 4 large organic egg whites 1¼ cups unsweetened almond milk
- 1 cup Cheddar cheese, shredded Ground black pepper, as required
- 2 tablespoons Parmesan cheese, shredded

DIRECTIONS

1. Preheat the oven to 350 degrees F (180 C. Grease a 9-inch pie plate.
2. In a skillet, melt the butter over medium heat and sauté the onion and garlic for about 2-3 minutes.
3. Add the broccoli and chicken and sauté for about 1-2 minutes.
4. Transfer the mixture into the prepared pie dish evenly.

5. In a bowl, add the eggs, egg whites, milk, cheddar cheese, salt and black pepper and beat until well combined.

6. Pour egg mixture over the chicken mixture evenly and top with Parmesan cheese.

7. Bake for about 40 minutes or until top becomes golden brown.

8. Remove from the oven and set aside for about 5 minutes before serving.

9. Cut into 8 equal sized wedges and serve.

NUTRITION: Net Carbs: 2.8g; Calories: 168; Total Fat: 8.5g; Sat. Fat: 4.2g; Protein: 18.8g; Carbs: 4g; Fiber: 1.2g; Sugar: 1.2g

Strawberry Cream Cheese Smoothie

Preparation Time: 5 minutes Cooking Time:

5 minutes Servings: 2

INGREDIENTS

- 1/4 cup fresh strawberries
- 1/2 tsp vanilla
- 1 tbsp butter, melted
- 1 cup heavy cream
- 3 oz cream cheese
- 1/2 cup ice

DIRECTIONS

1. Add all ingredients into the blender and blend until smooth and creamy.
2. Serve and enjoy.

NUTRITION: Calories 415 Fat 42.8 g Carbohydrates 4.3 g Sugar 1.2 g Protein 4.6 g Cholesterol 144 mg

Almond Butter Smoothie

Preparation Time: 5 minutes Cooking Time: 5 minutes

Servings: 1

INGREDIENTS

- 1 tbsp almond butter
- 1 tbsp unsweetened cocoa powder
- 2 cups unsweetened almond milk
- 5 drops liquid stevia

DIRECTIONS

1. Add all ingredients into the blender and blend until smooth and creamy.
2. Serve and enjoy.

NUTRITION: Calories 190 Fat 16.7 g Carbohydrates 9.9 g Sugar 0.8 g Protein 6.5 g Cholesterol 0 mg

Cocoa Sunflower Butter Smoothie

Preparation Time: 5 minutes Cooking
Time: 5 minutes Servings: 1

INGREDIENTS

- 1 tsp unsweetened cocoa powder
- 2/3 cup water
- 1/3 cup unsweetened coconut milk
- 2 tbsp sunflower seed butter
- 1/2 cup ice cubes

DIRECTIONS

1. Add all ingredients into the blender and blend until smooth and creamy.
2. Serve and enjoy.

NUTRITION: Calories 234 Fat 19.5 g Carbohydrates 11.8 g Sugar 0 g Protein 6.6 g Cholesterol 0 mg

Choco Peanut Butter Smoothie

Preparation Time: 5 minutes Cooking Time: 5 minutes Servings: 1

INGREDIENTS

- 1 scoop chocolate protein powder
- 5 drops liquid stevia
- 1 tbsp coconut oil
- 1 tbsp unsweetened cocoa powder
- 1 tbsp peanut butter
- 1/4 avocado
- 1/2 cup unsweetened coconut milk
- 3/4 cup unsweetened almond milk

DIRECTIONS

3. Add all ingredients into the blender and blend until smooth and creamy.
4. Serve and enjoy.

NUTRITION: Calories 379 Fat 31.1 g Carbohydrates 10.9 g Sugar 2.5 g Protein 16.3 g Cholesterol 20 mg

Refreshing Cranberry Smoothie

Preparation Time: 5 minutes

Cooking Time: 5 minutes Servings: 1

INGREDIENTS

- 1/5 cup cranberries
- 1 tbsp MCT oil
- 5 drops liquid stevia
- 1 cup unsweetened coconut milk

DIRECTIONS

1. Add all ingredients into the blender and blend until smooth and creamy.

2. Serve and enjoy.

NUTRITION: Calories 175 Fat 18 g Carbohydrates 7 g Sugar 2 g Protein 0 g Cholesterol 0 mg

Spinach Avocado Green Smoothie

Preparation Time: 5 minutes

Cooking Time: 5 minutes Servings: 1

INGREDIENTS

- 1/2 cup unsweetened coconut milk
- 1/4 tsp peppermint extract
- 1 scoop whey protein powder
- 8 drops liquid stevia
- 1 cup fresh spinach
- ½ avocado
- 1 cup ice

DIRECTIONS

1. Add all ingredients into the blender and blend until smooth and creamy.

2. Serve and enjoy.

NUTRITION: Calories 180 Fat 6.2 g Carbohydrates 7.4 g Sugar 1.2 g Protein 24 g Cholesterol 65 mg

3. **Rich & Creamy Blueberry** Smoothie

Preparation Time: 5 minutes

Cooking Time: 5 minutes Servings: 2

INGREDIENTS

- 1/2 cup blueberries
- 5 drops liquid stevia
- 1/2 tsp vanilla
- 1 tsp cinnamon
- 2 tbsp heavy cream
- 2 oz cream cheese
- 1 cup unsweetened almond milk

DIRECTIONS

1. Add all ingredients into the blender and blend until smooth and creamy.

2. Serve and enjoy.

NUTRITION: Calories 197, Protein 3.3 g Fat 17.3 g, Carbohydrates 8.5 g Sugar 3.8 g Cholesterol 52 mg

Easy Raspberry Smoothie

Preparation Time: 5 minutes

Cooking Time: 5 minutes Servings: 1

INGREDIENTS

- 1/2 cup raspberries
- 3/4 cup unsweetened almond milk
- 1/4 cup yogurt

DIRECTIONS

1. Add all ingredients into the blender and blend until smooth and creamy.

2. Serve and enjoy.

NUTRITION: Calories 90 Fat 3.6 g Carbohydrates 9.5 g Sugar 5.7 g Protein 4.6 g Cholesterol 4 mg

Mix Berry Breakfast Smoothie

Preparation Time: 5 minutes Cooking Time:
5 minutes Servings: 1

INGREDIENTS

- 1/4 cup frozen mixed berries
- 2/3 cup unsweetened almond milk
- 1 tbsp erythritol

DIRECTIONS

1. Add all ingredients into the blender and blend until smooth and creamy.

2. Serve and enjoy.

NUTRITION: Calories 65 Fat 4.1 g Carbohydrates 11.3 g Sugar 7.5 g Protein 0.3 g Cholesterol 0 mg

Healthy Carrot Smoothie

Preparation Time: 5 minutes Cooking Time: 5 minutes Servings: 2

INGREDIENTS

- 1 medium carrot, chopped
- 1 cup ice
- ¼ tsp nutmeg
- ¼ tsp cinnamon
- 8 drops liquid stevia
- 2 tbsp tahini
- 1/2 cup unsweetened coconut yogurt
- 1/4 cup unsweetened coconut milk

DIRECTIONS

1. Add all ingredients into the blender and blend until smooth and creamy.
2. Serve and enjoy.

NUTRITION: Calories 145 Fat 11.7 g Carbohydrates 10.2 g Sugar 2.2 g Protein 3 g Cholesterol 0 mg

Spicy Tuna Cups

Preparation Time: 5 minutes

Cooking Time: 25 minutes Servings: 6

INGREDIENTS

- 5 oz can tuna, drained
- 15 jar jalapeno slices
- 1 tbsp fresh parsley, chopped
- 1/2 cup pepper jack cheese, shredded
- 1/2 cup cheddar cheese, shredded
- 1/4 cup onion, chopped
- 1/4 cup mayonnaise
- 1/4 cup sour cream
- 2 eggs, lightly beaten
- Pepper
- Salt

DIRECTIONS

1. Preheat the oven to 350 F.
2. Spray a muffin tray with cooking spray and set aside.
3. In a large bowl, mix together eggs, parsley, cheese, onion, mayo, sour cream, tuna, pepper, and salt until well combined.
4. Pour egg mixture into the prepared muffin tray and top each

muffin cups with jalapeno slices.

5. Bake in preheated oven for 25 minutes.

6. Serve and enjoy.

NUTRITION: Calories 179 Fat 10.8 g
Carbohydrates 8.5 g Sugar 1 g Protein 11.3 g
Cholesterol 81 mg

Healthy Tuna Muffins

Preparation Time: 5 minutes Cooking Time: 25 minutes Servings: 8

INGREDIENTS

- 1 can tuna, flaked
- 1 tsp cayenne pepper
- 1 celery stalk, chopped
- 1 1/2 cups cheddar cheese, shredded
- 1/4 cup sour cream
- 1/4 cup mayonnaise
- 2 eggs, lightly beaten
- Pepper
- Salt

DIRECTIONS

1. Preheat the oven to 350 F.
2. Spray a muffin tray with cooking spray and set aside.
3. Add all Ingredients into the large bowl and mix until well combined and pour into the prepared muffin tray.
4. Bake in preheated oven for 25 minutes.
5. Serve and enjoy.

NUTRITION: Calories   188   Fat   13.9   g
Carbohydrates 2.6 g Sugar 0.7 g Protein 12.9 g
Cholesterol 75 mg

Chocolate Shake

Preparation Time: 5 minutes Cooking
Time: 5 minutes Servings: 1

INGREDIENTS

- 2 tbsp unsweetened cocoa powder
- 1/2 tbsp vanilla
- 1 1/2 tbsp hemp seeds
- 1 tbsp chia seeds
- 2 tbsp Swerve
- 2 tbsp almond butter
- 3/4 cup unsweetened almond milk
- 1/2 cup ice

DIRECTIONS

1. Add all Ingredients into the blender and blend until smooth and creamy.
2. Serve and enjoy.

NUTRITION: Calories 391 Fat 30.3 g
Carbohydrates 23.1 g Sugar 2.4 g Protein 15.1 g
Cholesterol 0 mg

Healthy Broccoli Mash

Preparation Time: 10 minutes Cooking Time:
5 minutes Servings: 6

INGREDIENTS

- 16 oz broccoli florets
- 1/2 tsp garlic, minced
- 1 tsp olive oil
- 1 tsp fresh lemon juice
- 1 cup of water
- Pepper
- Salt

DIRECTIONS

1. Add broccoli and water in a saucepan and cook over medium heat for 5 minutes. Drain well.
2. Transfer broccoli and remaining ingredients into the food processor and process until smooth.
3. Season with pepper and salt.
4. Serve and enjoy.

NUTRITION: Calories 33 Fat 1 g Carbohydrates
5.1 g Sugar 1.3 g Protein 2.1 g Cholesterol 0 mg

Mexican Cauliflower Rice

Preparation Time: 10 minutes Cooking Time:
15 minutes Servings: 4

INGREDIENTS

- 1 cauliflower head, chopped
- 1 tsp garlic powder
- 1 tsp chili powder
- 1 tsp cumin
- 1/4 cup tomatoes, diced
- 2 cups cooked chicken, shredded
- 1 tsp olive oil
- Salt

DIRECTIONS

1. Add cauliflower into the food processor and process until rice-sized pieces are formed.
2. Heat oil in a large pan over high heat.
3. Add cauliflower rice and chicken and cook for 5-7 minutes.
4. Add garlic powder, chili powder, cumin, tomatoes, and salt. Stir well and cook for 7-10 minutes more.

5. Serve and enjoy.

NUTRITION: Calories   141   Fat   3.6   g
Carbohydrates 5.1 g Sugar 2.1 g Protein 22   g
Cholesterol 54 mg

Healthy Collard Greens with Bacon

Preparation Time: 10 minutes Cooking Time: 8 minutes Servings: 4

INGREDIENTS

- 1 lb collard greens
- 1 tbsp apple cider vinegar
- 2 tbsp chicken broth
- 1/4 cup cherry tomatoes, halved
- 3 bacon slices, cooked and chopped
- 1 tbsp olive oil
- Pepper
- Salt

DIRECTIONS

1. Heat oil in a pan over medium heat.
2. Add collard greens, vinegar, broth, and tomatoes and cook for 6-8 minutes.
3. Add bacon and stir well. Season with pepper and salt.
4. Stir well and serve.

NUTRITION: Calories 142 Fat 10.3 g Carbohydrates 7 g Sugar 0.3 g Protein 8 g

Cholesterol 16 mg